THE AUTISM REVOLUTION

Unshackling the cause of Autism

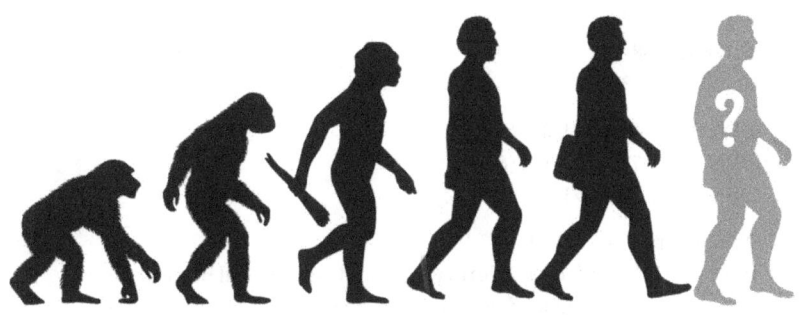

JOHN ETHERINGTON

First published 2025 by John Etherington

Produced by Independent Ink
independentink.com.au

Copyright © John Etherington

The moral right of the author to be identified as the author of this work has been asserted.

All rights reserved. Except as permitted under the *Australian Copyright Act 1968*, no part of this publication may be reproduced, stored in a retrieval system, or transmitted in any form or by any means, electronic, mechanical, photocopying, recording or otherwise, without prior written permission from the publisher. All enquiries should be made to the author.

Cover design by Catucci Design
Edited by Gail Tagarro from https://bookwritingcoach.com.au/
Internal design by Julian Mole at Post Pre-press
Typeset in 12/16 pt Adobe Text Pro by Post Pre-press Group, Brisbane

Cover image credits:
IS 1885694143
IS 178524048
IS 2205101363

ISBN 978-1-7642571-0-7 (Paperback)
ISBN 978-1-7642571-1-4 (epub)
ISBN 978-1-7642571-2-1 (Kindle)

Disclaimer:
This book is intended for informational and educational purposes only. It does not constitute medical, psychological, or therapeutic advice, nor is it intended to diagnose, treat, cure, or prevent any condition or disease. The content reflects the author's research, opinions, and lived experience and should not be interpreted as a substitute for professional consultation with a licensed healthcare provider. Readers are advised to seek appropriate professional guidance regarding any health-related concerns. Use of this book implies acceptance of this disclaimer.

To **Samantha**, whose strength, insight, and unwavering support have been the quiet force behind every step of this journey.

To **Eli**, whose curiosity and quiet strength inspire me to dream bigger and think deeper.

And to **Abby**, whose joy, imagination, and radiant spirit remind me daily of the beauty in being fully present.

You walked with me through every high and low, and helped turn this journey into something truly meaningful.

PREFACE

This book began with a question I couldn't ignore: Why do so many autistic individuals, despite their intelligence, insight, and capability, continue to be misunderstood, underutilized, and excluded from systems that claim to value diversity?

After my autism diagnosis in 2015, I began to reflect on a lifetime of challenges in education, employment, and navigating a world that often seemed to operate on rules I hadn't been given. Despite these challenges, I built a successful career in digital engineering and spatial science, eventually leading large-scale projects and managing teams of over 120 staff, with more than 80 autistic staff integrated into my team. In that role, I saw something that changed the course of my life: The problem wasn't autism. The problem was how the world was built to misunderstand it.

Even at the executive level, I encountered resistance, not just to new ideas but to new ways of thinking. I began to see a pattern: Autistic minds weren't failing to adapt to the world. The world was falling behind the autistic mind.

This realization led me to develop what I now call Mind Fidelity Theory, a framework that reimagines autism not as a deficit but as a different mode of perception and cognition. A mode that prioritizes accuracy over assumption, logic over social conformity, and truth over tradition. A mode that may be increasingly vital in a world defined by complexity, contradiction, and rapid change.

This book is the result of years of lived experience, professional leadership, and academic research. It is also a response to a growing call from researchers across disciplines for a unified, interdisciplinary theory of autism, one that integrates neuroscience, psychology, systems thinking, and lived experience. My current PhD research builds on this foundation, exploring cognitive modelling to investigate how communication and collaboration can be improved between individuals with varying levels of mind fidelity, particularly in the workplace. (Don't worry, I will explain mind fidelity in Chapter 1.)

What follows is not just a new theory about the origins of autism and the nature of autistic traits – it is a framework that seeks to identify their underlying cause. More than that, it is a new lens – one that I hope will help us see not only autism, but the entire human experience with greater clarity.

Let's begin.

CONTENTS

Chapter 1: The Puzzle Piece We've Been Missing — 1

Chapter 2: A History of Misunderstanding — 13

Chapter 3: Two Minds, One Reality — 18

Chapter 4: The Evidence for Mind Fidelity — 27

Chapter 5: The Biology of Mind Fidelity — 41

Chapter 6: Genetic Foundations of Autism — 52

Chapter 7: Evolution's Balancing Act – Complexity, Cognition, and the Rise of Autism — 64

Chapter 8: Theories of Autism Revisited – A Mind Fidelity Perspective — 75

Chapter 9: Diagnosis Reimagined – Behavior Through the Lens of Mind Fidelity — 89

Chapter 10: Leaving the Cave – Humanity's Next Step — 102

Final Summary: The Cause of Autism through Mind Fidelity Theory — 111

About the Author — 115

References — 117

CHAPTER 1: THE PUZZLE PIECE WE'VE BEEN MISSING

Imagine a young man named Alex. He's brilliant, a natural problem-solver, and deeply passionate about his education and work. But after graduation, something strange happens. Despite his qualifications, Alex struggles to find a job. When he does, it doesn't last. His colleagues misunderstand him. His managers say he's "too intense", "not a team player", or "missing the bigger picture". Eventually, Alex stops trying.

Alex is autistic, and his story is far from unique.

Across the world, autistic adults, especially those with higher education, face staggering rates of unemployment and underemployment.[1] In Australia, they have the highest unemployment rate of any disability group.[2] In the UK, only 15% of working-age autistic adults are in full-time employment,[3] and in the US, fewer than half are employed at all.[4]

This isn't because autistic people can't do the work. In fact, many are overqualified for the roles they're in. The problem lies elsewhere, somewhere deeper, more systemic, and more misunderstood.

The Inclusion Illusion

Over the past decade, companies have proudly embraced diversity and inclusion. They've brought in experts, hosted awareness days, and updated HR policies. But for autistic workers, these efforts often miss the mark. Despite accommodations and good intentions, the employment statistics for autistic adults have barely budged.[5]

Why?

Because most workplace interventions are built on a flawed assumption: That autistic people need to be "fixed" or "adjusted" to fit into a neurotypical world. The focus is solely on the autistic worker – through external accommodations, quiet rooms, flexible hours, and social skills training. While these are helpful, they don't address the root issue.

The real challenge isn't about noise sensitivity or eye contact. It's about how autistic and non-autistic people perceive the world, particularly how they reconstruct reality itself.

The Brain's Illusions

To understand this, we need to look at how the brain builds our experience of reality.

Have you ever felt your phone vibrate in your pocket, only to find it didn't? That's called phantom vibration syndrome,[6] and it's surprisingly common. Or consider the rubber hand illusion, where a person begins to feel ownership over a fake hand simply because it's stroked in sync with their real one.[7] These aren't just party tricks; they're profound demonstrations of how easily the brain can be tricked into believing something is real.

In both examples, the brain constructs a version of reality based on expectation, context, and internal models. Most of the time, we don't even notice. We just assume our experience is accurate because it feels real.

But what if some people, like those on the autism spectrum, experience less of this internal construction?

What if their brains rely more on direct external sensory input and less on internalized reconstruction?

This is the foundation of a new theory I call Mind Fidelity Theory.

Explaining The Terms

Mind Fidelity Theory describes how accurately the brain processes reality, and how this varies across individuals. It proposes that some minds construct much of their experience of internally, while others may rely more heavily on raw sensory input from the external world. This creates a spectrum: at one end, reality is shaped by internal models; at the other, it's anchored in objective truth. Illusions like phantom phone vibrations or the rubber hand effect show how convincing these internal constructions can be. Autistic individuals, however, may experience less interference from internal models – perceiving the world with higher fidelity to external reality. This isn't a flaw – though high levels of fidelity can present challenges – it's a different cognitive architecture and may just be the answer to what causes autistic traits.

What is Perception?
Perception is the gateway to reality. It's the process by which our senses detect and interpret the world around us – light, sound, texture, taste, and movement. Imagine standing in a forest: You hear birds singing, feel the breeze, and see sunlight filtering through leaves. These sensations don't just happen; your brain is actively constructing your experience from raw sensory input.

At its core, perception is about receiving and organizing information from the external world. It begins with sensation – what your eyes, ears, and skin detect – and continues as your brain filters, prioritizes, and gives meaning to that data. But perception isn't a perfect mirror. It's shaped by memory, expectation, and context. What we perceive is often what our brain expects to perceive.

What is Cognition?
Cognition is the mind's way of making sense of the world. It's the invisible engine behind everything we do when we think, learn, remember, or solve problems. Imagine your brain as a bustling city: Cognition is the traffic system, the power grid, and the communication network all rolled into one. It keeps ideas flowing, decisions moving, and memories lit up like neon signs.

Cognition builds on perception. It takes the raw sensory input we receive and begins to organize, evaluate, and respond to it. When we recognize a friend's face, solve a puzzle, or plan a conversation, we use cognitive skills like attention, memory, reasoning, and language. It's not just about being "smart"; it's about how we interpret signals from the world and respond in meaningful ways.

What is Fidelity?
Most of us will recognize the word fidelity as connected to actions in marriage; however, in the science of measurement, fidelity has a different meaning.

Fidelity is the measure of how accurately something reflects or reproduces its original form. It's a concept that shows up in many fields – technology, science, design, and even storytelling – and it always points to the same idea: Staying true to the source.

In audio and video, fidelity refers to the quality of reproduction. For example, high-fidelity sounds mean the audio you hear is very close to the original performance; clear, detailed, and undistorted. If you've ever listened to music on a high-end speaker system and felt like the band was right there in the room with you, that's high fidelity in action. On the other hand, a low-fidelity recording might sound muffled or scratchy, losing much of the richness and nuance of the original.

In design and engineering, fidelity describes how closely a model or prototype matches the final product. A high-fidelity prototype of a smartphone, for instance, might include a working touchscreen, realistic weight, and functioning apps, ideal for testing user experience. A low-fidelity prototype, by contrast, might be a simple sketch or a cardboard mock-up, useful for early brainstorming but not for detailed testing.

Fidelity also plays a role in data transmission and simulation. In digital communications, signal fidelity refers to how accurately data is transmitted from one point to another without distortion or loss. In simulations, like flight training or virtual reality, high-fidelity environments aim to replicate real-world conditions as closely as possible, providing a more immersive and reliable experience.

In all these cases, fidelity is about accuracy. It's the standard by which we judge how well something captures the essence of what it's meant to represent.

A New Theory Emerges

As described above, Mind Fidelity Theory suggests that humans process reality on a spectrum, weighted by a balance of raw veridical perceptions (truth-aligned to external reality), and internally created perceptions. In this framework, autistic individuals process external reality with a higher degree of accuracy, or "fidelity". Unlike most people, who often simplify complex information by relying on cognitive shortcuts known as biases and heuristics, autistic individuals may be less influenced by these internal filters. While such shortcuts can make everyday decision-making more efficient, they also introduce distortions that reduce the minds fidelity to an external objective reality.

A central idea in Mind Fidelity Theory is that coherence, or the ability to perceive and interpret reality in a way that aligns with a social unit, increases as mind fidelity decreases. In other words, when perception is less anchored to raw external sensory input, and the mind filters and fills in gaps using internalized interpretations shaped by social expectations and experiences, social cohesion increases, but at the cost of fidelity to objective reality. This process creates a shared, socially cohesive version of reality, but one that is less objectively accurate.

As with many cognitive traits, balance is key. Mind Fidelity Theory proposes that either extreme – too much or too little fidelity – can lead to significant challenges. At very high levels of fidelity, a person may become overwhelmed by unfiltered sensory or perceptual input, making it difficult to generalize, interpret context, or engage fluidly with the social world.

This heightened sensitivity can interfere with the ability to link sensory information, such as spoken language, to relevant memories for understanding. As a result, speech development may be delayed in childhood, a characteristic often observed in individuals on the autism spectrum.

Conversely, when fidelity is too low, perception and cognition may become dominated by internal projections rather than external reality, potentially contributing to phenomena such as hallucinations, as seen in conditions like schizophrenia.

An Extension of Dual Processing

Mind Fidelity Theory builds on the well-established Dual Process Theory[8] that suggests humans have two modes of thinking:

- Type 1: Fast, intuitive, automatic, driven by experience and expectation.
- Type 2: Slow, deliberate, analytical, driven by logic and evidence.

Most people default to Type 1 thinking.[9] It's efficient and socially cohesive. But it's also prone to error, especially in complex or unfamiliar situations. Research suggests that autistic individuals tend to favor Type 2 thinking.[10] They question assumptions, resist social framing, and prioritize accuracy over conformity.

This difference isn't just academic; it has real-world consequences. In a workplace built on intuition, hierarchy, and unspoken norms, someone who values logic over social cues can be seen as difficult, disruptive, or even disabled.

But what if they're not?

What if they're simply seeing the world more accurately, less filtered by bias, and more grounded in reality?

The Unshackled Prisoner

To explore this idea, let's expand on one of the oldest philosophical metaphors, Plato's Allegory of the Cave.

In it, prisoners are chained in a cave, watching shadows on the wall, believing them to be reality. One prisoner is taken out of the cave, sees the world as it truly is, and then returns, only for their revelation to be rejected by those still in chains.

This book argues that autistic individuals are, in many ways, the unshackled prisoners of our time. They see the world differently, not incorrectly but more accurately (what is casting the shadows, rather than the shadows themselves). And in a society built on shared illusions, beliefs, and filtered reality, that difference is often punished rather than celebrated.

What This Book Explores

Over the coming chapters, we'll delve into:

- The history of autism and the limitations of current theories
- The cognition and neuroscience of perception and how reality is constructed by the mind
- The genetic and evolutionary forces that may be shaping human cognition
- An elaboration of Plato's Allegory of the Cave, revealing its relevance to modern cognitive and perceptual diversity.

- The answer to the question that has puzzled scientists for generations: What causes autism?

This is not just a book about autism. It's a book about how we think, how we evolve, and how we build a future that works for all minds. Through an interdisciplinary exploration of neuroscience, genetics, cognition, and lived experience, it follows the evidence to uncover the underlying cause of autism and autistic traits. It will unify our understanding of what autism is, why it exists, and why its prevalence is increasing at an extraordinary pace.

CHAPTER 2: A HISTORY OF MISUNDERSTANDING

Autism has always been here, but how we've understood it has changed dramatically over time.

From Schizophrenia to Spectrum

The word "autism" was coined in 1911 by Swiss psychiatrist Eugen Bleuler to describe one of the several types of schizophrenia: A withdrawal from reality. For decades, children who today would be recognized as autistic were instead diagnosed with childhood psychosis or schizophrenia.[11]

It wasn't until the 1940s that two researchers, working independently, began to describe something different. In the United States, Leo Kanner observed a group of children who seemed socially withdrawn but intellectually capable. He called it "early infantile autism". Around the same time in Austria, Hans Asperger described children with similar traits – an intense focus, unusual communication styles, and deep knowledge in specific areas. His work would later inspire the term Asperger's Syndrome.[12]

Still, it took until 1980 for autism to be formally recognized in the Diagnostic and Statistical Manual of Mental Disorders (DSM-III).[13] Even then, it was narrowly defined. Over time, the criteria expanded and in 2013, the DSM-V edition introduced the term we use today: Autism spectrum disorder (ASD), a broad umbrella that acknowledges the wide range of traits and abilities among autistic individuals.[14]

The Deficit Model

For most of its history, autism has been framed as a deficit, a list of things a person can't do. Can't make eye contact, can't understand social cues, can't adapt to change, etc. This view has shaped everything from education to employment to therapy. It has also shaped how autistic people see themselves.

Three major theories have emerged to explain these perceived deficits.

1. Theory of Mind (ToM): The idea that autistic people struggle to understand that others have thoughts and feelings different from their own.[15]
2. Weak Central Coherence: The idea that autistic people focus too much on details and miss the "big picture".[16]
3. Executive Dysfunction: The idea that autistic people have trouble with planning, flexibility, and self-regulation.[17]

Each of these theories captures part of the picture, but none of them has succeeded in explaining the whole spectrum of behavior.

A Shift in Perspective

In recent years, a new wave of research has begun to challenge the deficit model. One of the most important ideas is the Double Empathy Problem, proposed by Damian Milton.[18] It suggests that communication breakdowns between autistic and non-autistic people are mutual, not the fault of one side. In other words, it's not that autistic people lack empathy; it's that both groups struggle to understand each other's way of thinking.

This shift has opened the door to strength-based approaches, focusing on what autistic people do well rather than what they lack. But even these newer models often fall short. They still operate within a framework that assumes neurotypical thinking is the norm and everything else is a variation.[19]

What if that assumption is wrong?

The Need for a New Framework

As we've seen, the history of autism is a history of misunderstanding. From schizophrenia to spectrum, from deficit to difference, we've been inching closer to a more accurate view, but we're not there yet.

What's missing is a theory that explains not just the behaviors of autistic individuals but the cognitive architecture behind them. A theory that accounts for both the challenges and the strengths. A theory that recognizes autism not as a disorder but as a natural variation in how the brain processes reality.

That's where Mind Fidelity Theory comes in.

In the next chapter, we explore the science behind how humans think, and how we make decisions, form beliefs, and construct our sense of reality. We'll begin to see why autistic minds may not be broken at all but rather tuned to a different frequency.

CHAPTER 3: TWO MINDS, ONE REALITY

Every day, we make thousands of decisions, like what to eat, how to respond to a colleague, and whether to trust a stranger. Most of these decisions happen without us even realizing it. We just "know". But how do we know?

Cognitive science tells us that the human brain operates using two distinct systems of thought. As mentioned in the previous chapter, this is known as Dual Process Theory, and it has become one of the most influential models in psychology.

The Two Systems

Type 1 thinking is fast, automatic, and intuitive. It's the gut feeling you get when something seems off.

It's the snap judgment you make in a conversation. It's efficient, emotional, and shaped by experience.

Type 2 thinking is slow, deliberate, and analytical. It's what you use when solving a complex math problem, planning a strategy, or questioning your own assumptions. It takes effort, but it's also more accurate.

Most people rely heavily on Type 1 thinking. It's what allows us to navigate social situations, make quick decisions, and function in a complex world without constant mental overload. But as mentioned earlier, it's also prone to bias.[9]

Confirmation bias
Confirmation bias is the tendency to seek out, interpret, and remember information in a way that supports what we already believe. Instead of objectively weighing all evidence, we often give more attention to data that confirms our views, and we ignore or downplay anything that contradicts them. For example, someone who believes a particular diet is the healthiest might only read articles that praise it while dismissing studies that highlight its risks. This bias can reinforce misconceptions and make it harder to change our minds, even in the face of strong evidence.

Authority bias

Authority bias occurs when we place too much trust in the opinions or instructions of someone perceived as an authority, regardless of the actual quality or relevance of their input. This can happen in classrooms, workplaces, or in advertising. For instance, a person might accept a medical claim simply because it was made by someone in a lab coat, even if that person isn't a qualified expert. While respecting expertise is often useful, authority bias can lead us to overlook critical thinking or alternative perspectives.

Halo effect

The halo effect is a mental shortcut where our overall impression of a person, brand, or idea influences how we judge their specific traits. If someone is physically attractive or well-spoken, we might also assume they're intelligent, kind, or competent, even without evidence. For example, a charismatic speaker might be seen as more trustworthy, even if their arguments are weak. This bias can shape hiring decisions, product reviews, and even courtroom outcomes, often without us realizing it.

Some other biases of note that readers may choose to explore are anchoring bias, optimism bias, negativity bias, framing effect, Dunning-Kruger effect, illusion of control, gambler's fallacy, sunk cost fallacy, belief bias, attentional bias, and the bandwagon effect. While this is not a comprehensive list, it provides an example of how much of what we perceive as real is simply an illusion.

The Benefit of Bias

Mind Fidelity Theory proposes that cognitive biases are not simply flaws or quirks of the human mind, but rather evolved adaptations shaped by natural selection. These mental shortcuts may have developed because they enhanced social cohesion and group survival.

In ancestral environments, individuals who aligned their perceptions and beliefs with those of the group were more likely to be accepted, protected, and supported. Over time, this tendency to prioritize social harmony over strict perceptual accuracy may have offered a survival advantage, especially in larger, cooperative groups. In this view, biases are not just errors; they are features of a mind optimized for navigating complex social environments.

As will be discussed in detail later, evolutionary simulations, such as those presented in the paper *Natural Selection and Veridical Perceptions*, offer compelling support for this idea.[20]

These simulations demonstrate that organisms that perceive reality with high accuracy (veridically) are often outcompeted by those whose perceptions are less accurate but more strategically useful. In the simulated environments, the organisms that interpret the world in ways that maximize survival and reproduction, regardless of whether those interpretations reflect objective truth, are more likely to thrive. This suggests that evolution may favor utility of the mind (the most useful perception and cognition of reality) over accuracy of the mind (the perceptions that are a true reflection of reality), reinforcing the idea that cognitive biases and heuristics are not simply mental errors, but adaptive strategies shaped by the demands of survival.

While Type 1 thinking – fast, intuitive, and automatic – has long served as the backbone of human survival, Type 2 thinking introduces a slower, more deliberate mode of reasoning. It allows for abstract thought, long-term planning, and the evaluation of complex, hypothetical scenarios.

Though more cognitively demanding, Type 2 thinking is closely associated with higher mind fidelity. It enables individuals to override instinctive biases and heuristics in favor of more accurate, reflective judgments. From an evolutionary perspective, this mode of thinking may have initially emerged as a rare but advantageous trait, gradually gaining utility as human societies became more complex.

This shift can be understood through the lens of the evolutionary process of stabilizing selection,[21] where traits that balance adaptability and efficiency are favored over extremes. In early environments, high-fidelity perception and cognition may have been costly, too slow, or too socially disruptive to be advantageous. However, as human environments became increasingly more complex and shaped by technology and information access, the ability to think abstractly and model reality with greater accuracy became more valuable. Type 2 thinking, once a cognitive luxury, began to offer real survival and social advantages.

This transition is echoed in Grinin's Curve,[22] a model that describes the accelerating pace of human development. This is described in more detail in Chapter 7. The curve illustrates how technological and societal complexity has grown, not linearly but hyperbolically, with each innovation laying the groundwork for faster and more transformative changes.

As humans created tools, language, agriculture, and eventually digital systems, the demands on our cognitive systems increased. In this context, the utility of high-fidelity perception and cognition, supported by Type 2 thinking, has grown in parallel with the complexity of our environments.

Thus, Mind Fidelity Theory suggests that the evolutionary balance between Type 1 and Type 2 thinking is not fixed but dynamic. As our environments become more abstract and interconnected, the selective pressures may increasingly favor minds capable of higher fidelity processing, potentially contributing to the rising prevalence of autistic traits in newer generations.

This idea will be explored in greater depth in Chapter 7, where we examine how modern challenges may be reshaping the perceptual and cognitive balance toward higher fidelity.

The Cost of Clarity

At first glance, this might seem like a superpower. Who wouldn't want to be more rational, less biased, more accurate?

But there's a catch.

Our social world is built on shared assumptions, emotional cues, and unspoken rules, all shaped by Type 1 thinking and reinforced by cognitive shortcuts.

These heuristics help people navigate complex social environments quickly and with minimal effort. When someone doesn't play by those rules, when they prioritize truth over politeness or logic over social convention, they can be seen as cold, awkward, or difficult, even if they're technically right.

This is the paradox at the heart of autism in the modern world: Greater mind fidelity – encompassing both perceptive and cognitive accuracy – can lead to greater social friction.

The question then becomes: Is autism the deficit, or is it simply the signal of evolution?

Mind Fidelity Theory invites us to consider that autistic traits are not flaws to be corrected but indicators, early warnings that our current social, political, and organizational systems may no longer be well suited to the complexity of the environments we've created. As our world becomes more abstract, interconnected, and information-dense, the utility of a high-fidelity mind increases. Yet, many of our institutions remain optimized for a world that rewards conformity, intuition, and fast, low effort thinking.

To treat autism as a problem to be fixed rather than as a message to be understood is to risk ignoring a vital alarm. In systems theory, this is known as signal suppression, when a system silences or disregards feedback that could help it adapt. History shows that ignoring such signals can lead to collapse, stagnation, or crisis. If we continue to pathologize the minds that are best adapted to our environment's emerging complexity, we may be blinding ourselves to the very insights we need to evolve our societies.

A Different Kind of Mind

In later chapters, we'll explore how this difference in perception and cognitive processing plays out in real-world situations, especially in the workplace. We'll see how autistic individuals often clash with systems designed for intuitive thinkers, and how this clash can be misunderstood as a deficit rather than a difference.

But first, we'll take a closer look at the evidence, the studies, the neuroscience, and the patterns that support this new way of understanding the autistic mind.

CHAPTER 4: THE EVIDENCE FOR MIND FIDELITY

If autistic individuals really do process the world differently – not less effectively but more accurately – then we should be able to see it in the data, and we do.

Across multiple domains of psychology and neuroscience, a consistent pattern emerges. Autistic minds tend to favor logic over intuition, evidence over assumption, and external reality over internal narrative.

Let's explore what cognitive science research tells us.

Reasoning: When Logic and Belief Collide

One of the most revealing ways to understand how people think is by looking at how they reason, especially when logic and belief point in different directions.

Take this example.

> All flowers need water.
> Roses need water.
> Therefore, roses are flowers.

At first glance, the conclusion feels right. Roses are flowers, after all. But here's the twist: The logic doesn't hold up.

Why? Because the conclusion doesn't logically follow the premise. The first statement tells us something about all flowers. The second tells us something about roses. However, it was never established that roses are part of the flower group. The structure is flawed, even if the conclusion happens to be true in real life.

This is a classic example of what psychologists call belief bias; our tendency to accept arguments that align with what we already believe, even if the reasoning is faulty. When the conclusion feels true, we're more likely to overlook whether the logic is sound.

But here's where it gets interesting. Research shows that people with high autistic traits are less likely to fall into this trap. They're more inclined to focus on the structure of the argument itself rather than on how believable the conclusion seems. In other words, they're more likely to say, "Wait a minute, this doesn't logically follow," despite knowing that roses are flowers. [23]

This suggests a more substantial reliance on Type 2 thinking, a slower, more deliberate form of reasoning that checks our gut instincts. Most of us rely heavily on Type 1 thinking, shaped by our beliefs and experiences. But Type 2 thinking is what helps us step back and ask, "Does this actually make sense?"

So, when logic and belief collide, many of us go with what feels right. But those who are less swayed by belief, like many autistic individuals, may be better equipped to spot the flaw. It's not about being smarter; it's about processing information differently.

Decision-Making: Clearer Thinking, Fewer Biases

When it comes to making decisions, most of us are influenced by more than just facts. Emotions, social expectations, and the way information is presented can all shape our choices, often without us even realizing it.

However, research shows that autistic individuals often approach decisions differently. They tend to be less swayed by emotion or social framing and more focused on logic and consistency.[24]

Take the Ultimatum Game, for example. In this experiment, the first player offers to split a sum of money with another. The second player can accept the offer or reject it, but if they reject it, neither player gets anything. Most people reject offers they see as unfair, even if it means walking away with nothing. It's an emotional response: "That's not fair, so I won't take it."

However, autistic participants are more likely to accept the offer if it makes rational sense, like getting $2 instead of $0, even if it feels unfair. Their decisions are guided more by outcome than emotion.[24]

This pattern shows up in other areas, too. In studies on framing effects, people are asked to choose between options that are logically identical but worded differently. For instance, would you prefer a surgery with a "90% survival rate" or one with a "10% mortality rate"? Most people choose the first, even though both mean the same thing. The wording changes how it feels.

Autistic individuals, however, tend to see through this framing. They're more likely to recognize that the two options are equivalent, refraining from changing their decision based on how the information is presented.[24]

This kind of clear, consistent thinking shows up across many types of decisions by autistic minds.[24]

Less sunk-cost bias: They're less likely to keep investing in something just because they've already spent time or money on it.

Less optimistic bias: They don't assume that good outcomes are more likely just because they hope for them.

More stable choices: Even in emotionally charged or uncertain situations, their decisions tend to be more consistent and less reactive.

This doesn't mean autistic individuals are emotionless or robotic. It means that they often process information in a more analytical way, especially when others are swayed by feelings or social pressure. It's a different cognitive style, one that can lead to more rational and reliable decisions.

Metacognition: Confidence Without Overconfidence

One of the more subtle but powerful differences in how autistic individuals think lies in metacognition, the ability to reflect on one's own thinking. It's not just about making decisions, but about how confident we are in those decisions and whether that confidence is justified.

Research shows that autistic individuals often display lower initial confidence in their judgments compared to their non-autistic peers. But here's the key: Their confidence tends to align more closely with reality. They're less likely to be overconfident and more likely to adjust their certainty based on evidence and feedback. In other words, they're not second-guessing themselves out of insecurity; they're calibrating their confidence to match the facts.[25]

This stands in contrast to a common cognitive bias seen in many people: Overconfidence. In many settings, especially high-stakes environments like business or leadership, confidence is often mistaken for competence. And that can lead to costly errors in judgment.

A Workplace Analogy

Imagine a group of executives at a fast-growing tech company. They've just hired a new salesperson – let's call him Jake – who walks into the boardroom with charisma, a firm handshake, and a dazzling pitch. He speaks with conviction, drops buzzwords effortlessly, and projects absolute certainty in his strategies.

The team is impressed. Jake's confidence is contagious. Within weeks, he's led strategy meetings, been asked for input on product direction, and is praised for his "leadership potential". His ideas, though often vague or inconsistent with industry best practices, are rarely questioned. This is a classic example of the halo effect, where one positive trait (in this case, confidence) colors how we perceive everything else about a person.

But one executive isn't convinced.

Sitting quietly at the end of the table is Maya, an autistic executive known for her analytical thinking and attention to detail. She's noticed that Jake's proposals lack substance. His numbers don't add up. His strategies contradict established data. She raises these concerns, pointing out inconsistencies and asking for clarification.

But her feedback is brushed aside. "You're overthinking it," someone says. "Jake knows what he's doing."

Maya doesn't push back emotionally. She simply continues to gather evidence, document discrepancies, and refine her analysis. Her confidence in her concerns grows, not because she feels more certain, but because the data supports her conclusions. Still, the team remains under Jake's spell, interpreting the alarm as a battle of egos.

The Risk of Overconfidence and the Value of High Mind Fidelity

In the above example, Jake isn't intentionally misleading anyone. His overconfidence is genuine, and that's precisely the problem. Overconfidence, especially when paired with social biases like the halo effect, can distort group decision-making. When confidence is mistaken for competence, organizations become vulnerable to poor choices, missed risks, and costly missteps.

This scenario also highlights a deeper issue: Autistic individuals are often blamed for social breakdowns, for being "too blunt", "too rigid", or "not a team player". In reality, it is often their loyalty to truth, accuracy, and cognitive integrity that challenges the social norms others take for granted. Maya isn't being disruptive; she is being diligent. Her commitment to evidence over ego should be seen as an asset, not a liability.

In a world where groupthink and charisma can overshadow substance, organizations would do well to recognize the value of minds like Maya's. Autistic thinking may not always align with social expectations, but it often aligns more closely with reality. And in business, as in life, that's what ultimately matters.

This alignment with reality isn't just philosophical; it's cognitive. The same traits that make autistic individuals less susceptible to social biases also equip them with unique problem-solving strengths. Their ability to focus intensely, think systematically, and perceive patterns others might miss becomes especially powerful when tackling complex, abstract challenges.

Problem-Solving: Visual Strengths and Systematic Thinking

When faced with complex problems, especially those that require spotting patterns or thinking abstractly, autistic individuals often perform in ways that challenge traditional expectations. Their strengths in visual reasoning and systematic analysis can lead to faster, more accurate solutions, particularly on tasks that don't rely heavily on verbal or social reasoning.

One striking example comes from studies using Raven's Progressive Matrices,[26] a well-known test of abstract reasoning. It's designed to measure fluid intelligence, the ability to solve new problems without relying on prior knowledge. In these studies, autistic participants often score significantly higher than their measured IQ predicts. Not only do they solve the problems more accurately, but they do so more quickly, suggesting they are using a different cognitive strategy, one that emphasizes structure, logic, and visual pattern recognition over intuition or verbal reasoning.

This raises an intriguing question: What kind of thinking is at play here?

Type 1 vs. Type 2 Thinking: A Quick Primer

As discussed earlier, psychologists often divide thinking into two different modes, Type 1 and Type 2.

In the general population, access to Type 2 thinking is often linked to IQ.[9] People with higher IQs tend to have more cognitive resources available to engage in this slower, more effortful mode of reasoning. But here's where things get interesting.

Autistic Thinking: A Different Route to Type 2

Studies suggest that autistic individuals may have greater access to Type 2 thinking, even when their measured IQ is average or below average. In other words, they may be more likely to engage in deliberate, logical reasoning regardless of IQ level. This challenges the traditional view that access to Type 2 thinking is purely a function of intelligence.[27]

Instead, it suggests a distinct cognitive architecture – one that prioritizes accuracy over speed, structure over intuition, and logical reasoning over social cues. This may reflect a biological divergence, where autistic cognition embodies a more direct and generalized access to Type 2 thinking (deliberate, analytical thought), bypassing the conventional developmental pathway typically associated with high intelligence.

This perspective helps explain why autistic individuals often excel in fields that require systematic analysis, such as mathematics, engineering, computer science, and design. Their minds are naturally tuned to detect inconsistencies, follow rules, and solve problems in a methodical way.

Rethinking Cognitive Strengths

Too often, autistic perception and cognition is framed in terms of deficits or what it lacks compared to neurotypical norms. But when we look at how autistic individuals approach problem-solving, a different picture emerges: One of high perceptive and cognitive fidelity, logical accuracy, and visual–spatial strength.

Rather than being a limitation, this style of thinking may offer unique advantages, especially in a world that increasingly values data, systems, and innovation. It also invites us to rethink how we define intelligence and success, not just in academic settings but in workplaces, communities, and society at large.

Putting it all Together: The Cognitive Signature of Autism

Across the domains we've explored – reasoning, decision-making, problem-solving, and metacognition – a consistent and compelling pattern emerges: Autistic individuals tend to process information with greater mind fidelity.

As proposed by the Dual Process Theory of Autism, they are less influenced by internal biases, more grounded in external reality, and more consistent in their logic. They show a preference for structure over assumption, evidence over intuition, and accuracy over social harmony. This doesn't mean they're always right or that they don't face challenges. But it does mean that their minds are tuned differently, not broken, not deficient, but often more aligned with the structure of reality than with the social consensus around it.

What's particularly striking is that many of these strengths, such as enhanced access to Type 2 thinking, suggest that autistic cognition may represent a distinct cognitive architecture, one that prioritizes analytical reasoning and perceptual accuracy as a baseline mode of processing.

This reframes autism not as a deficit in social cognition but as a different mode of cognition altogether, one that may have evolved to serve different adaptive purposes.

But if this cognitive style is truly distinct, then we must ask: Can we see it in the brain?

Looking Ahead: From Cognition to Neuroscience

If autistic individuals think differently, then those differences should be reflected not just in behavior but in biology. Increasingly, neuroscience is beginning to reveal just that.

In the next chapter, we'll explore how these cognitive traits, such as heightened pattern recognition, reduced bias, and analytical consistency, may be rooted in the structure and function of the brain. We'll look at how differences in sensory processing, neural connectivity, and brain region activation may help explain the unique strengths of autistic cognition.

By bridging the gap between how autistic individuals think and how their brains are wired, we can begin to build a more complete and scientifically grounded understanding of autism, not as a disorder of deficits but as a neurocognitive identity with its own strengths and its own place in the human story.

CHAPTER 5: THE BIOLOGY OF MIND FIDELITY

If autistic individuals think differently, then those differences must be rooted in something more profound than behavior, something biological. After all, cognition doesn't happen in a vacuum. It emerges from the brain: A living, dynamic system shaped by evolution, experience, and sensory input.

In the previous chapter, we explored how autistic individuals often show a distinct cognitive profile, one marked by logical accuracy, reduced bias, and a consistent preference for evidence over assumption. These traits suggest a different mode of processing the world, one that may not rely on intuition or social cues in the same way neurotypical cognition does.

But where do these differences come from?

To answer that, we need to look beneath the surface into the neuroscience of autism. If increased perceptual and cognitive fidelity to objective reality is a defining feature of autistic thinking, then we should expect to find its fingerprints in the structure and function of the brain itself.

In this chapter, we'll explore how differences in sensory processing, neural connectivity, and brain region activation may help explain the unique cognitive strengths of autistic individuals. We'll look at how the brain's wiring supports a heightened sensitivity to detail, a preference for patterns, and a resistance to social and emotional bias.

And we'll ask a deeper question still. Could these neurological differences represent not a disorder but an alternative design, a different way of being human, with its own strengths and its own evolutionary purpose?

Let's begin where cognition starts, with the senses.

Reception and Transduction: The Sensory Gateways

Perception begins with sensation. Before the brain can interpret the world, it must first detect it and then translate it. This two-step process starts with reception, where specialized sensory receptors in the eyes, ears, skin, nose, and tongue respond to physical stimuli like light, sound, smell, pressure, and chemicals. It continues with transduction, where these stimuli are converted into electrical signals the brain can understand.

In autistic individuals, this system often functions differently. Research shows that sensory input may be either heightened or diminished, not due to preference but because of biological differences in receptor sensitivity and signal processing.[28] A flickering light that goes unnoticed by one person might feel painfully intense to another. A soft fabric might feel abrasive, or a background hum might dominate attention.

These differences extend into transduction. Neuroimaging studies suggest that the autistic brain may process sensory signals with greater intensity or altered timing. This can lead to sensory distortions, where sounds seem sharper, lights brighter, or touch more intense. These aren't hallucinations but rather a different prioritization of sensory data, which can sometimes result in altered sensation.[29]

In essence, the autistic sensory system may be tuned to a different frequency, one that captures more raw detail but also risks overload.

Transmission: The Brain's Wiring

After sensory signals are converted into electrical impulses, they must travel through the brain's intricate network of neurons to reach the appropriate processing centers. This stage, called transmission, is like a relay race, where information is passed from one neuron to the next across complex pathways.

Neuroimaging studies have shown that autistic individuals often exhibit distinct patterns of neural connectivity. One common finding is increased local connectivity (how well nearby brain regions communicate) with stronger and denser connections within specific brain regions.[30] At the same time, long-range connectivity (involving communication between distant areas of the brain) is often reduced.

These patterns are not uniform across all autistic individuals. The degree and location of these connectivity differences can vary widely, reflecting the diversity of the autistic population. Some individuals may show pronounced differences in sensory regions, while others may exhibit variations in areas related to attention, memory, or motor control. Yet others with ASD show long-range overconnectivity.[30]

What is clear is that the architecture of the autistic brain is measurably different from that of neurotypical individuals. Whether these differences are inherently better or worse is context dependent. However, what is key to our understanding is that they are distinct and understanding them is a crucial step toward appreciating the full range of human neurodiversity.

Perception: Constructing Reality

Perception is not a passive process. It is an active construction shaped by how the brain filters, prioritizes, and integrates sensory information. At the center of this process lies the thalamus, a deep brain structure often described as the brain's "sensory relay station". All sensory input except smell passes through the thalamus before reaching the cortex, where it is interpreted and given meaning.

Neuroimaging studies have revealed that autistic individuals often show unusual patterns of connectivity between the thalamus and various cortical regions. Two key findings stand out:[31]

- Hyperconnectivity between the thalamus and the temporal lobe. This region is involved in processing auditory information, language, and

aspects of social cognition. Increased connectivity here may reflect heightened sensitivity to sensory input, or differences in how auditory and social information is processed.
- Reduced connectivity between the thalamus and the prefrontal cortex. The prefrontal cortex is associated with executive functions such as planning, decision-making, and emotional regulation. Weaker connections in this pathway may influence how sensory information is integrated with higher-order cognitive processes.

These findings suggest that the thalamus may play a central role in shaping the perceptual experiences of autistic individuals. Importantly, the patterns of connectivity are not uniform across all autistic people. There is considerable variability, reflecting the diversity of the spectrum.

Perception involves both bottom-up and top-down processing. Bottom-up processing is driven by raw sensory data, while top-down processing relies on prior knowledge, expectations, and memory.[32]

In neurotypical individuals, top-down processing often dominates. The brain uses past experiences to interpret incoming sensory data, filling in gaps and smoothing over inconsistencies. This is efficient, but it also introduces bias. What we perceive is not always what is there; it is often what the brain expects to be there based on experience.

In autistic individuals, research suggests that bottom-up processing may play a more significant role. Reduced connectivity between sensory regions and memory-related areas means that less prior knowledge may be used to filter incoming data, resulting in a more raw, unfiltered experience of the world.[32]

But what does memory have to do with filtering sensory information?

Filtering Reality: Processing Limits, Memory, and Cognitive Bias

The human brain is constantly flooded with sensory information, far more than it can consciously process. To manage this overload, it relies on filtering mechanisms that prioritize certain inputs while discarding others. This isn't a flaw; it's a feature. But it also means that what we perceive is not a perfect mirror of reality. Rather, it is a curated or recreated version shaped by what the brain deems important.

One of the most powerful tools the brain uses to filter information is memory. Past experiences help the brain decide what to pay attention to and what to ignore. This makes perception faster and more efficient, but it also introduces bias.

A relatable example of this is what often happens when you buy a new car. Suddenly, you may start seeing the same make and model everywhere: On the road, in parking lots, at traffic lights. It's not that everyone else has bought the same car. Those cars were always there. But before, the brain didn't assign them any special meaning, so they were filtered out. Now that the car has personal relevance, the brain includes it in conscious perception.

This shift is a perfect example of top-down processing, where memory and meaning influence what we notice.

This mechanism may have evolved to help us prioritize information that's relevant to our goals, safety, or identity. Once something becomes meaningful, whether it's a car, a face, or a potential threat, the brain begins to treat it as important. It becomes part of the "approved" sensory stream, while less relevant data is rejected, or it fades into the background.

However, this same system that helps us draw consistent perceptions of our reality can also lead to cognitive bias. Because the brain tends to notice what it expects or values, it can overlook or dismiss information that doesn't fit with existing beliefs. This is how belief bias and cognitive dissonance arise.[33] When new information challenges what we already "know", the brain may resist it, not because it's wrong, but because it's unfamiliar or inconsistent with our previous experiences.[34]

In this way, perception is not just about what enters our senses; it's about what our brain allows us to see.

This filtering effect can also be seen in the workplace. Take an employee, for example, trained to perform a specific task, who may unconsciously ignore information that falls outside the scope of their training. Their perception becomes streamlined and efficient but narrow. In contrast, an autistic employee, who may not rely as heavily on learned expectations or who may be less impeded by selective filtering, might notice details others overlook.

For example, while a team is focused on following a standard procedure, the autistic individual might detect a subtle inconsistency in data, a pattern in customer feedback, or a flaw in a system that others have filtered out. Not because they are smarter or more intelligent, but because their brain didn't reject the information as irrelevant through selective filtering.

In this way, autistic perception can serve as a kind of cognitive safety net, catching what others miss.

Autism and the Filtering of Sensory Information

In autistic individuals, research suggests there may be reduced connectivity between sensory regions and memory-related areas of the brain, such as the medial prefrontal cortex.[31] This could mean that less prior knowledge is used to filter incoming data, resulting in a more raw, unfiltered experience of the world.

Where a neurotypical person might walk into a room and immediately tune out the hum of a refrigerator, an autistic person might hear it clearly and continuously because their brain isn't filtering it out.

This may also explain why autistic individuals are often less susceptible to visual illusions or social expectations. They are not filling in the gaps with assumptions or excluding new sensory data based on internalized beliefs to the same extent.

A Different Kind of Perception

Rather than reconstructing a version of reality based on memory and belief, the autistic brain may be more likely to perceive what is actually present, even if it's overwhelming or socially unexpected. This can lead to a perception that is less biased, more detailed, and more grounded in the immediate sensory environment.

Conclusion: A Different Kind of Mind

From the receptors in the skin to the circuits of the brain, the autistic sensory system is not broken; it's different. These differences can lead to challenges, but they also offer unique strengths: Heightened attention to detail, resistance to bias, and a commitment to truth over comfort.

Understanding these biological foundations helps us see autism not as a deficit but as a distinct cognitive style, one that may offer a clearer, more objective view of reality in a world clouded by illusion.

In the next chapter, we delve into the genetic foundations of autism, exploring what could be causing these biological differences.

CHAPTER 6: GENETIC FOUNDATIONS OF AUTISM

Autism is often described in terms of behavior, how someone communicates, interacts, or responds to the world. But beneath those behaviors lies something deeper: Biology. And at the heart of that biology is genetics.

In this chapter, we explore the genetic foundations of autism, not as a list of mutations or medical terms but as a story about how the brain is built. We'll look at how certain genetic changes shape the systems responsible for perception, and how these changes may lead to a different way of experiencing the world.

Rather than viewing these differences as flaws, we'll consider them as part of a broader pattern, one that may reflect an ongoing shift in how human minds are evolving. From spontaneous mutations to ancient regions of DNA that evolved rapidly in humans, the genetics of autism may hold clues not just to how autistic brains work, but also to how all human cognition is changing.

Let's begin by looking at one of the most intriguing sources of genetic variation: De novo mutations.

De Novo Mutations: New Instructions for Building the Brain

Sometimes, a person is born with a genetic change that neither parent carries. These are called de novo mutations, which simply means "new mutations". They happen spontaneously during the earliest stages of development, like a new instruction written into the blueprint of the brain.

These mutations don't follow a single pattern. Instead, they tend to show up in a wide variety of genes. But what many of these genes have in common is this: They help build the biological systems that shape how we perceive the world.

Let's explore how these systems work.

The Brain's Wiring System

The brain is made up of billions of neurons, and synapses are the tiny junctions where these neurons connect and communicate. Think of them as the wiring that allows signals to travel from one part of the brain to another.

Genes involved in synaptic function help determine how these connections form, how strong they are, and how efficiently they transmit information. When de novo mutations affect these genes, it can lead to differences in how sensory signals – like sights, sounds, and textures – are processed and interpreted.

Opening the Right Pages

Inside every cell, DNA is tightly packed and organized. However, for a gene to be used, it needs to be accessible. Chromatin remodeling is the process that opens up the DNA so the cell can read the right instructions at the right time.

Mutations in genes that control this process can influence which parts of the brain develop more actively, how neurons grow and connect, and how responsive they are to sensory input. These changes can subtly reshape the architecture of perception: How the brain receives and organizes information from the outside world.

Managing the Blueprint

Once the DNA is accessible, the cell needs to copy the instructions and carry them out. This process is called transcription, and it's tightly regulated. Genes involved in this step act like managers, deciding which instructions get used, when, and how much.

When mutations affect these regulatory genes, it can shift the timing and balance of brain development. This can influence how sensory systems mature, how they prioritize different types of input, and how they interact with memory and attention systems.

A Different Way of Seeing

What ties all this together is that these genetic changes, though varied and complex, tend to influence the biological foundations of perception. They don't just affect one part of the brain. They shape the systems that determine how we experience the world from the very beginning: How we hear, see, feel, and interpret what's around us.

In autism, these changes may lead to a brain that is tuned differently; not broken, but built with a different set of priorities, a brain that may process more raw sensory data and organize it in ways that don't rely as heavily on experience or expectation.

We'll explore what this means in the next chapter, where we look at how evolution may favor these kinds of changes, not as errors but as part of a broader process of adaptation and balance.

Copy Number Variations: Extra or Missing Pieces

Sometimes, sections of DNA are accidentally duplicated or deleted. These are called copy number variations, or CNVs. Think of them as having extra pages, or missing pages, in the instruction manual for building the brain.

When these changes happen in genes that are involved in brain development, they can affect how the brain's sensory systems are wired. This might influence how sensitive someone is to sound, how they process visual information, or how they respond to touch.

In autism, CNVs are more common than in the general population.[35] And while each variation is different, many of them seem to affect the parts of the brain that help us take in and make sense of the world. These changes don't just alter behavior; they shape the biology of perception and cognition itself.

Common Genetic Variants: Small Changes, Big Patterns

Not all genetic differences are rare or dramatic. Some are small, common variations that many people carry. On their own, they might not have much effect. But when many of them appear together, they can subtly shift how the brain develops and functions.

In autism, these common variants often show up in genes that influence how neurons grow, connect, and communicate, especially in areas of the brain involved in sensory processing and attention.[36]

It's like adjusting the settings on a camera. Each change is small, but together, they can create a very different picture. These subtle shifts may lead to a brain that processes the world with a different rhythm or focus, one that's more tuned to raw sensory input and less shaped by expectation.

Gene Networks: Systems that Shape the Senses

Genes don't work alone. They operate in networks, groups of genes that interact to build and maintain the brain's structure and function. Some networks are especially important for perception. They help form synapses, regulate how genes are turned on and off, and guide the development of sensory pathways.

In autism, many of the genes that show differences belong to these networks. This suggests that the changes aren't random; they're clustered in systems that shape how we experience the world.

When these networks are altered, the result may be a brain that organizes sensory information differently. It might be more sensitive to detail, more focused on patterns, or less influenced by experience. These are not flaws; they are variations in how perception is built from the ground up.

Gender Differences: Different Thresholds, Same Foundations

Autism is more commonly diagnosed in males than females. This has led researchers to suggest that females may have a kind of biological "buffer", requiring a higher threshold of change before traits become noticeable. Nevertheless, when females are diagnosed, they often carry more significant genetic changes.[37]

What's important here is that the same kinds of genetic changes, whether in males or females, often affect the same systems – those involved in perception, attention, and sensory regulation.

This means that while the expression of autism may differ between genders, the underlying biology often points to the same foundations. It's not about one group being affected either more or less; it's about how different brains respond to the same kinds of changes in the systems that shape how we see, hear, and feel the world.

Human Accelerated Regions: The Fast Lane of Human Evolution

Imagine a part of the human genome that's racing ahead of the rest, evolving faster, changing more rapidly, and shaping what it means to be human. These are human accelerated regions or HARs.

Discovered in 2006, HARs are stretches of DNA that have remained relatively unchanged across millions of years of evolution, until humans came along.[38]

In our species, these regions suddenly took off, evolving at a pace far beyond the rest of the genome. What makes this even more fascinating is where these changes are happening – not just in the genes that build muscles or bones, but also in the ones that help build the brain.

HARs don't typically code for proteins themselves. Instead, they mostly act like genetic switches, turning other genes on or off, especially during early brain development. They help guide how neurons grow, how they connect, and how different regions of the brain communicate. Interestingly, HAR 1, the fastest accelerating HAR, directly affects the development of the cortex region of the brain,[38] the area responsible for accepting or rejecting the raw sensory data sent by the thalamus, ultimately determining our perception of reality.

Recent research has also shown that HARs are especially active in neurons, the cells responsible for processing and transmitting information in the brain. This suggests that HARs may play a key role in shaping how we perceive, interpret, and respond to the world around us.

A Double-Edged Blueprint

But evolution doesn't always move in a straight line. The same regions that may have helped humans develop complex thought and language can also be sites of vulnerability. Variations in HARs have been found in individuals with autism spectrum disorder (ASD) and schizophrenia,[39] two conditions that, while very different, both involve changes in how the brain constructs reality.

In autism, these variations may contribute to a brain that is more tuned to external reality and less influenced by social expectations or internal bias. In schizophrenia, the opposite may occur: A brain that becomes overly shaped by internal narratives, sometimes at the expense of what's there in reality.

This contrast opens a fascinating possibility: That HARs are not just about making us human, they may also be part of what makes human perception so diverse. They may influence the balance between bottom-up sensory input and top-down interpretation, shaping how much we rely on raw data versus internal models in perceiving reality.

A Theory of Mind Fidelity

This is where Mind Fidelity Theory comes in. The theory proposes that autistic individuals process the world with greater fidelity to external reality, less filtered by bias, assumption, or social framing. If HARs are part of the machinery that builds this perceptual system, then variations in HARs could help explain why some minds are more anchored in what is, while others are more influenced by what is expected.

Rather than seeing these variations as errors, Mind Fidelity Theory suggests they may be part of an ongoing evolutionary process, one that is still shaping how humans think, perceive, and adapt.

Summary

In this chapter, we explored the genetic foundations of autism, focusing on how various genetic changes influence the biology of perception. We looked at de novo mutations, copy number variations, common genetic variants, gene networks, and gender differences, all of which shape how the brain processes sensory information.

We then delved into human accelerated regions (HARs), unique to humans, evolving rapidly, and playing a crucial role in brain development and cognitive function. These regions may contribute to the diversity of human perception, influencing the balance between how much external sensory input we process in balance to what we internally create.

Mind Fidelity Theory proposes that these genetic variations are not errors but part of an ongoing evolutionary process, enhancing fidelity to external reality in autistic individuals. This theory suggests that autism represents a different way of processing the world, one that prioritizes accuracy over social conformity.

In the next chapter, we will explore how evolution may favor these kinds of changes, not as errors, but as part of a broader process of adaptation and balance.

CHAPTER 7: EVOLUTION'S BALANCING ACT — COMPLEXITY, COGNITION, AND THE RISE OF AUTISM

A New Question Emerges

In the previous chapter, we explored the genetic foundations of autism and how spontaneous mutations, copy number variations, and rapidly evolving regions of the human genome known as human accelerated regions (HARs) may shape how autistic individuals perceive the world. But this raises a deeper question.

What could be causing these genes to change in the first place?

Why would evolution favor traits that lead to a radically different way of thinking that resists social conformity, filters less, and clings more tightly to objective reality?

To answer this, we need to zoom out. Way out. We must look at the entire arc of human development, not just biologically but socially, culturally, and cognitively.

From Tribes to Technology: Humanity's Expanding Complexity

The human story begins in small, tightly knit tribal groups. In these early communities, survival depended on social cohesion. Trust, shared beliefs, and synchronized behavior were not luxuries but lifelines. A tribe that was fractured over disagreements, or that failed to act in unison during a hunt or a threat, would not survive.

In this context, the human brain evolved to prioritize social harmony over objective truth. Minds that could quickly align with the group by filtering out conflicting information, reinforcing shared beliefs, and trusting authority were more likely to survive and reproduce. These cognitive shortcuts – biases and heuristics – became embedded in our psychology. They helped us navigate a dangerous world by simplifying it, and as humanity grew, so did our environment.

Tribes became villages, villages became cities, cities became nations, and now, we live in a globalized world where every belief system, culture, and ideology is just a click away.

With each leap in scale, the complexity of our environment increased. And with it, the demands on our cognition.

Grinin's Curve: Mapping the Acceleration of Human Development

Russian historian and economist Professor Leonid Grinin proposed a model of human development that helps us understand this acceleration.[22] Known as Grinin's Curve, it suggests that human progress doesn't move in a straight line; it moves in stages, each subsequent one shorter and more intense than the last.

Take the invention of the wheel. At first, it was a simple tool. But it enabled farming and increased transportation, which led to food surpluses, population growth, and cities. Cities brought new challenges, like sanitation, governance, trade, and conflict. Each solution created new problems, and each problem demanded more complex thinking.

This is the essence of Grinin's Curve; each innovation increases the complexity of the environment, which demands more of the human mind.

Now, we've entered the Information Age. Unlike the wheel, which changed how we move, the internet has changed how we think. Information is no longer passed down slowly through generations; it's instant, global, and overwhelming. Competing ideas are everywhere. Long-held beliefs are constantly challenged. And the old cognitive tools – biases, heuristics, and social conformity– are starting to show their limits.

This is the new complexity. And it may be the most significant turning point in the human story.

Stabilizing Selection: Nature's Balancing Act

To understand how evolution responds to this complexity, we turn to a concept called stabilizing selection.

Stabilizing selection is an evolutionary process that favors traits that strike a balance, traits that are just right for the environment. It weeds out extremes that are too far in either direction.[21]

But stabilizing selection doesn't just apply to physical traits. It also applies to cognition.

The Science of Variation and Evolutionary Extremes

In evolutionary biology, variation is not a flaw; it's a feature. Every population, whether of birds, bacteria, or humans, contains a range of traits. This range is not random; it's the result of genetic recombination, mutation, and environmental pressures. Stabilizing selection acts on this variation by favoring traits that are most adaptive to the current environment, while filtering out those that are too far from the optimal range.

However, evolution doesn't eliminate extremes entirely. In fact, it relies on them. These outliers, individuals with traits far from the average, serve as a kind of biological experiment, constantly testing the boundaries of what might be useful in a changing world. This is a well-documented phenomenon in evolutionary theory: Populations maintain a low but persistent frequency of extreme traits, which can become advantageous if the environment shifts.

This principle is supported by evolutionary game theory and simulation models, where populations are shown to maintain a distribution of traits that includes rare, high-risk, high-reward strategies. These outliers may not thrive in the current environment, but they are evolution's hedge against uncertainty, a way of preparing for future conditions that might favor a different kind of mind or body.

Making it Real: The Spectrum of Perception

Now, let's bring this back to human cognition.[40]

Imagine a spectrum of how humans perceive reality. On one end are minds that interpret the world almost entirely through internal filters – social expectations, cultural norms, and cognitive shortcuts like confirmation bias. These minds are highly efficient in stable, familiar environments. They prioritize coherence and consensus, which helps maintain social harmony.

On the other hand, there are minds that perceive the world with high fidelity to external reality. These individuals rely less on internal models and more on raw sensory input. They are less influenced by social framing and more attuned to inconsistencies, patterns, and objective data. This kind of perception can be socially disruptive, but it can also be highly adaptive in complex or novel environments.

Most people fall somewhere in the middle. But evolution always produces variation. Some individuals, outliers, are born with extreme traits. These outliers may struggle in the current environment, or they may be early indicators of where evolution is heading.

In the context of Mind Fidelity Theory, these outliers may represent a shift in the balance of perception from socially cohesive but biased cognition to more accurate, less filtered cognition. As our environment becomes more complex, interconnected, and information-dense, the utility of these high-fidelity minds to the environment increases.

They are not errors. They are experiments. And in the grand narrative of evolution, they may be the prototypes of the future.

Seeing What Matters: The Utility of Perception

To explore this further, let's look at the work of cognitive scientist Donald Hoffman. Hoffman and his team ran thousands of evolutionary simulations in virtual environments. In these simulations, organisms competed for survival. Some could see all of reality, some could see part of it, and some could see none of it, only what was useful for survival.[20]

The results were surprising; the organisms that saw none of the reality, only what was relevant to their fitness, outcompeted those that saw more of reality. In other words, evolution doesn't favor truth; it favors utility.

This means our success as a species doesn't necessarily mean we perceive reality accurately. Instead, our brains use shortcuts and adaptations – mental "tricks and hacks" – to shape our perception in ways that help us navigate and survive in our environment. This requires a mind that is designed to be adaptive, that helps us survive, not one that helps us understand truth or reality.

But what happens when the environment becomes so complex that the old tricks no longer work?

What happens when success in the environment requires more accuracy/fidelity to objective reality and less bias?

Mind Fidelity and the New Evolutionary Pressure

As the environment becomes more complex socially, technologically, and informationally, the utility of high-fidelity perception and cognition increases. Minds that can resist bias, question assumptions, and process raw data without distortion become more valuable.

This shift is not random. It's evolutionary.

Grinin's Curve shows us that human development is accelerating. Stabilizing selection tells us that evolution favors traits that are best suited to the current environment. Mind Fidelity Theory proposes that autistic traits, such as bottom-up processing, analytical reasoning, and resistance to social framing, are increasingly adaptive in this new world.

Autism, then, is not a disorder to be fixed. It is a signal, a sign that the human mind is evolving through adaptation to meet the demands of a more complex environment.

Looking Ahead: Mind Fidelity Theory and Autism

As we've explored throughout this chapter, the increasing complexity of our environment may be driving evolutionary changes in how the human mind processes reality. Mind Fidelity Theory offers a compelling framework for understanding these changes, not just as abstract shifts in cognition, but as tangible traits that are becoming more visible in the population, particularly through the lens of autism.

Rather than viewing autism as a disorder or developmental disability, this theory invites us to see it as a natural variation in cognitive architecture, one that may be better suited to the demands of a rapidly evolving world, but inconsistent with our current structure. The traits we associate with autism may not be flaws to be corrected but early adaptations that reflect a deeper fidelity to external reality, a reduced reliance on the social filters and cognitive shortcuts that once served us well in simpler times.

In the next chapter, we'll explore how Mind Fidelity Theory can help us make sense of the many behaviors, diagnostic criteria, and long-standing theories that have shaped our understanding of autism. By reinterpreting these through the lens of fidelity, we may begin to see a more unified, coherent picture, one that not only explains the past but also points toward a more inclusive and insightful future.

CHAPTER 8: THEORIES OF AUTISM REVISITED – A MIND FIDELITY PERSPECTIVE

For decades, autism has been explained through a series of psychological theories. These models, while insightful, often framed autism as a collection of deficits or deviations from what is normal. But what if there is no normal?

In this chapter, we'll revisit the major theories of autism and explore how the new framework of Mind Fidelity Theory can unify and reframe them.

The Theory of Mind

ToM suggests that autistic individuals struggle to understand that others have thoughts, feelings, and perspectives different from their own.[41] This idea emerged in the 1980s when researchers noticed that many autistic children had difficulty with tasks requiring them to imagine what someone else might believe or feel. This led to the concept of "mind-blindness".

Mind Fidelity Theory, however, suggests that autistic individuals may not be "mind blind" but rather, less influenced by the social illusions that shape neurotypical thinking. If your brain is wired to prioritize truth over assumption, it may not automatically simulate what others believe, especially if those beliefs are based on social conventions or experience. It's not a lack of empathy, but a different way of processing social information. This has been highlighted in the double empathy problem raised by an autistic academic, Damian Milton, which we will explore a bit later in this chapter.

Weak Central Coherence

Weak central coherence (WCC) proposes that autistic people tend to focus on details at the expense of the "big picture". This idea emerged from observations that autistic individuals often excel at tasks involving patterns, fine details, or local features but may struggle with tasks that require integrating information into a broader context, like understanding the overall theme of a story or interpreting social nuance.[42]

From the perspective of Mind Fidelity Theory, this detail-focused style is not a flaw; it's a feature. Autistic individuals may be less likely to "fill in the gaps" with assumptions, prior beliefs, or social expectations. Instead, they see what is actually there, not what they expect to see. This can make it harder to interpret ambiguous or socially constructed situations, but it also allows for extraordinary accuracy, pattern recognition, and insight into systems that others might overlook.

Interestingly, even the originators of this theory have challenged the idea that it reflects a deficit. Uta Frith, who first proposed WCC, later remarked, "This is so ironic because I use it to celebrate the children's strengths. It's not good always to be taken in by the whole: this means you have prejudices, and it weakens independent thought."[11] Similarly, Simon Baron-Cohen, a leading autism researcher, has said, "I don't go along with the term 'weak' in weak central coherence. It implies something that is underdeveloped, whereas if you look at the tests Uta does, the individuals often show strengths. Children with autism are often very good at seeing patterns."[11]

These reflections reinforce the idea that what has long been seen as a limitation may, in fact, be a strength, one that offers a clearer, more objective view of reality. In a world increasingly shaped by complexity and abstraction, the ability to see the parts before the whole may not only be valuable but essential when there is an abundance of information.

Executive Dysfunction Theory

Executive Dysfunction Theory suggests that autistic individuals may struggle with planning, flexibility, and self-regulation, skills collectively known as executive functions. This idea emerged from observations that autistic people often have difficulty switching tasks, adapting to change, or organizing their thoughts in ways that align with typical expectations.[17]

In classrooms, this might look like a student who becomes distressed when the schedule changes unexpectedly. In the workplace, it might be an employee who excels at deep, focused work but finds it challenging to juggle multiple shifting priorities.

Traditionally, these behaviors have been interpreted as signs of dysfunction, evidence that something is impaired or underdeveloped. However, Mind Fidelity

Theory offers a different explanation. It suggests that autistic individuals often operate with a high degree of cognitive fidelity, meaning they rely more on deliberate, logical processing, what psychologists call Type 2 thinking, as previously discussed.

The trade-off is that Type 2 thinking demands more cognitive resources, particularly working memory.[9]

When a person is already using much of their mental bandwidth to process information, which would traditionally be processed by Type 1 thinking, there's less capacity left for rapid task-switching or spontaneous adaptation. It's not that the person can't be flexible, but that the cognitive capacity required for flexibility is competing for resources already at capacity. Such conscious shifts in focus would not only be more difficult for someone with higher cognitive fidelity but would also be frustrating and draining.

Imagine trying to write a detailed report while someone keeps changing the topic mid-sentence. Or picture a chess player being asked to switch games every few moves, each with a different set of rules. That's what it can feel like for a high-fidelity mind navigating a world built for fast, intuitive thinkers. The same deep focus that enables analytical brilliance can make rapid shifts more difficult, not because of a flaw but because of the depth of processing involved.

This perspective reframes executive challenges not as deficits but as the natural consequence of a different cognitive architecture. In fact, what looks like rigidity may be consistency. What appears as inflexibility may be a commitment to accuracy. And what's often labelled as disorganization may simply be a mismatch between how the mind works and how the environment expects it to behave.

Understanding this trade-off allows us to move beyond the language of dysfunction. It invites us to see autistic cognition not as broken but as optimized for a different kind of task, one that values depth over speed, logic over instinct, and truth over convenience.

Social Motivation Theory

Social Motivation Theory suggests that autistic individuals are less driven by the desire for social interaction.[43] This idea emerged from observations that autistic children often showed less interest in faces, avoided eye contact, or preferred solitary play over group games. In traditional developmental psychology, these behaviors were interpreted as signs of social disinterest or even emotional detachment.

But what if that interpretation is incomplete?

Mind Fidelity Theory offers a different lens. It proposes that the autistic brain may not automatically assign value to social cues in the same way a neurotypical brain does, not because it lacks empathy or interest but because it isn't biased by the same social expectations.

In most people, social signals like a smile, a raised eyebrow, or a subtle tone shift are instantly and unconsciously prioritized. These cues are loaded with meaning, not because they are inherently important, but because our brains have been trained, through experience, to treat them as such.

For someone with high perceptive and cognitive fidelity, however, that automatic prioritization doesn't happen. Their brain doesn't assume that a smile means friendliness or that eye contact is necessary for connection. Instead, they may focus on the literal content of what's being said or on the logic of a conversation rather than the emotional subtext. This doesn't mean they don't care; it means they're processing the interaction based on analysis rather than intuition and experience.

Imagine a child who prefers to line up toy trains by color and size rather than join a game of pretend tea party. To an outside observer, this might look like social withdrawal. But to the child, the trains offer a world of structure, logic, and clarity, qualities that social interaction often lacks. Or consider an adult who avoids small talk at work but lights up when discussing a shared interest in astronomy or computer programming. Their connection is real; it's just built on shared knowledge rather than shared emotion or belief.

Autistic individuals may seek connection through mutual interests, deep conversations, or collaborative problem-solving. They may not be drawn to social rituals like birthday parties or networking events, but they often form strong, loyal bonds with those who understand and respect their way of relating.

In this light, the so-called "lack" of social motivation isn't a deficit; it's a difference in what is perceived as meaningful. It's not that autistic people don't want to connect. It's that they may be navigating a world where the usual social currency – eye contact, small talk, and emotional mirroring – don't hold the same value. When we recognize that, we can begin to build bridges based on mutual understanding rather than misinterpretation.

Enhanced Perceptual Functioning

Enhanced Perceptual Functioning (EPF) theory suggests that autistic individuals often excel at processing raw sensory information – what scientists call "low-level perceptual abilities". These are the brain's most basic ways of detecting and responding to sights, sounds, textures, and other sensory input before any conscious thought or interpretation takes place. For example, someone might notice tiny differences in patterns, hear faint background noises others miss, or detect subtle changes in light or texture. These abilities reflect a cognitive style that's finely tuned to detail and precision, often prioritizing accuracy over generalization.[44]

Mind Fidelity Theory builds on this by proposing that autistic minds process the world with less internal filtering and more direct access to external reality. In most people, the brain acts like a compression algorithm; it filters out what it deems irrelevant, fills in gaps based on experience, and smooths over inconsistencies to create a coherent, simplified version of reality. This is efficient, but it comes at a cost; important details may be lost, and assumptions may override accuracy.

By contrast, autistic individuals may experience the world with fewer of these filters. Their perception is less shaped by expectation and more grounded in what is present. They don't just notice more; they notice what others miss.

Imagine walking into a room and instantly hearing the faint hum of a fluorescent light, feeling the subtle texture of the carpet underfoot, and spotting a crooked picture frame on the wall. While others might tune out these details, the autistic mind may register them all with equal clarity. This heightened perceptual fidelity can be overwhelming at times, but it also enables a level of awareness and insight that is often extraordinary.

In practical terms, this can translate into remarkable abilities in fields that require accuracy and pattern recognition, such as mathematics, music, engineering, or design. It can also mean noticing inconsistencies in data, errors in code, or subtle shifts in tone that others might miss. These are not just quirks; they are cognitive strengths.

Rather than viewing enhanced perception as a side effect of autism, Mind Fidelity Theory positions it as a core feature. It's a different way of engaging with the world, one that values accuracy over assumption and detail over generalization. In a society that often rewards speed and simplification, this kind of thinking may be underappreciated. But in a world that increasingly depends on managing complexity, nuance, and innovation, it may be exactly what humans need to adapt.

The Double Empathy Problem

The Double Empathy Problem argues that social misunderstandings between autistic and non-autistic people are mutual, not the fault of one side. Damian Milton proposed that autistic people don't lack empathy; they just experience and express it differently.[18] Mind Fidelity Theory supports the idea that both groups operate with different cognitive systems, one based on social coherence and the other on perceptual accuracy, leading to mutual misunderstanding. It's not a deficit. It's a difference in how reality is constructed.

Mind Fidelity: The Common Thread in a Spectrum of Difference

While each of the major theories of autism – ToM, Weak Central Coherence, Executive Dysfunction, Social Motivation, and Enhanced Perceptual Functioning – has contributed valuable insights, none has been able to fully explain the wide range of autistic traits.[45] Each theory captures a piece of the puzzle, but they all fall short of offering a universal framework.

One reason for this is the inconsistencies observed across individuals on the spectrum. Some autistic people show strong executive functioning, while others struggle. Some are highly socially engaged, while others are withdrawn. Some excel in pattern recognition, while others do not. These variations have long puzzled researchers and clinicians alike.

Mind Fidelity Theory offers a unifying explanation, not only for the strengths and challenges described by these theories but also for the inconsistencies between them. It does so by framing autism as a product of evolutionary variation. In this view, autism is not a single condition, but a spectrum of cognitive architectures shaped by evolutionary forces.

Evolution does not produce uniform outcomes. It experiments. It generates variation, billions of small genetic and neurological differences, each unique, in an ongoing attempt to find the most adaptive traits for a given environment. In the case of autism, this means that different individuals may have different biological configurations. Some may have heightened auditory sensitivity; others enhanced visual processing; some may rely more on bottom-up sensory input; and others may show reduced social filtering. These differences are not random; they are part of a broader evolutionary strategy to explore new ways of perceiving and interacting with an increasingly complex world.

This is why autism is not consistent. That is why it exists on a spectrum. This is why the behaviors and traits associated with autism can vary so widely. But despite this variation, one pattern emerges repeatedly: An increased fidelity to objective reality. Whether it manifests as a resistance to social framing, a preference for logic over intuition, or a heightened sensitivity to sensory input, the autistic mind tends to process the world with greater accuracy and less distortion. It is this fidelity to external reality, this reduced reliance on internal bias and assumption, that unites the autistic spectrum.

Mind Fidelity Theory doesn't just explain what autism is. It explains why it looks different in every person. It also shows us that behind the diversity of traits lies a consistent cognitive signature, a mind tuned more closely to what is and less to what is expected.

A Diagnostic Approach

As we've seen, Mind Fidelity Theory not only reframes the evidence of the major theories of autism but also explains the inconsistencies that have long puzzled researchers. It offers a unifying lens through which the diversity of autistic traits begins to make sense, not as a flaw in the theories but as a reflection of the evolutionary variation that shapes human perception and cognition itself.

But understanding autism isn't just about theory. It's also about how we recognize it in the real world, how we define it, diagnose it, and describe the behaviors that bring it into focus.

In the next chapter, we'll explore the diagnostic criteria for autism and the traits most associated with it. And we'll ask, if autism is a spectrum, what exactly is varying? How does Mind Fidelity Theory help us make sense of that variation?

Let's turn now to the lived experience of autism, the patterns, the behaviors, and the spectrum that connects them all.

CHAPTER 9: DIAGNOSIS REIMAGINED — BEHAVIOR THROUGH THE LENS OF MIND FIDELITY

Autism is diagnosed through observable behaviors, but these behaviors are often misunderstood. Traditional models interpret them as deficits, considering them failures for not meeting neurotypical norms. Mind Fidelity Theory offers a different view: These traits are not flaws but reflections of a mind more in tune with reality that prioritizes accuracy over assumption and logic over social convention. Disability, then, should not be defined by deviation from the majority, but by how well a cognitive profile aligns with the demands of its environment.

Let's explore how this theory reframes the diagnostic landscape through real-world scenarios.

A Child's Experience

Imagine a young child in school. This child might struggle with social interactions, finding it difficult to make eye contact or engage in small talk. Traditional theories might label these behaviors as deficits in social communication. However, Mind Fidelity Theory offers a different lens. It explains why this child's brain doesn't automatically assign meaning to social signals. Due to increased perceptive and cognitive fidelity, the child's focus is on the literal content of what's being said or on the logic of a conversation rather than the emotional subtext. This doesn't mean they don't care; it just means they're processing things differently.

As mind fidelity increases, so does the brain's commitment to Type 2 processing – deliberate, analytical, and resource intensive. But this comes at a cost. Working memory becomes heavily taxed, leaving fewer cognitive resources available for Type 1 processes, which are fast, intuitive, and often socially directed. In this high-fidelity state, the brain prioritizes correctness and logic over heuristics and cognitive shortcuts. It aims to replicate reality more accurately, rather than filtering and adapting it to previous experience and belief.

The Yin and the Yang

This trade-off has profound implications for social behavior. Making eye contact, for example, is a behavior often loaded with social meaning, yet it varies widely across cultures. In some societies, eye contact is seen as a sign of respect or engagement, and neurotypical children typically learn this through repeated social reinforcement. They internalize it without conscious effort.

However, for individuals with high mind fidelity, the story is different. Their brains prioritize literal information and logical consistency over socially constructed cues. As a result, eye contact doesn't automatically carry the same weight or value. Instead, it becomes a conscious, effortful task, something that must be deliberately managed. And because their cognitive resources are already heavily taxed by processing the world with perceptive accuracy, maintaining eye contact can feel intrusive or overwhelming. In this context, reduced eye contact isn't a sign of disinterest or avoidance; it's likely a strategy to reduce cognitive load and protect an already overburdened mind.

As mind fidelity increases along the spectrum of human cognition, the ability to conform to social and behavioral norms may diminish. This is not due to a lack of desire or empathy but rather to the reallocation of cognitive resources. The brain is so finely tuned to logical consistency and literal interpretation that it bypasses the associative, emotionally nuanced pathways that facilitate intuitive social behavior, not out of dysfunction or desire but because these pathways are assigned lower priority in the brain's allocation of processing resources. While to a neurotypical individual, social behavior is valued, to an autistic mind, it is not relevant to reality. Therefore, the cognitive cost is not prioritized.

In contrast, as mind fidelity decreases along the spectrum of human cognition, there may be a greater reliance on Type 1 thinking. This increases the value of social expectations and allows for more fluid, intuitive social interactions, albeit sometimes at the expense of objective truth. Individuals with less extreme increases in fidelity levels may exhibit more socially normative behavior, but this behavior may still be consciously adopted rather than deeply internalized.

The Disruptive Student

In another example, consider an adolescent in high school. This student might excel in subjects like mathematics, physics, or computer science, where accuracy, logic, and structured problem-solving are rewarded. These subjects align well with higher levels of mind fidelity, which favors literal interpretation, rule-based reasoning, and deep focus. However, the same student might struggle in other subjects that rely on social conditioning – such as English, history, drama, religious studies, and social studies – destroying their motivation and self-worth and leading to overall reduced grades.

Where Weak Central Coherence Theory might suggest that this student is "missing the big picture" in such subjects mentioned above due to a detail-focused cognitive style, Mind Fidelity Theory offers a different interpretation.

The student isn't failing to see the big picture; they're seeing what is there, unfiltered by social assumptions or emotional expectations. This clarity, however, can create friction in subjects that reward socially conditioned interpretations. When asked to analyze a character's motives or a historical event, the student may return an answer that is logically consistent but lacks the emotional framing or social nuance the teacher expects. In some cases, their response may even be misinterpreted as insensitive or inappropriate, not because it is hateful, but because it challenges the socially accepted narrative.

While such answers may be marked incorrect, they are not signs of misunderstanding. They are expressions of a mind that values objective accuracy over social precision. If truth is defined by social consensus rather than logical coherence, then a high-fidelity mind will naturally resist that consensus, not out of defiance, but out of commitment to what it perceives as real.

In this context, the student's difficulty with abstract or socially interpretive subjects is not a deficit but a byproduct of a high-fidelity perceptive and cognitive system that prioritizes accuracy over inference. The trade-off is clear: Greater analytical accuracy at the cost of reduced intuitive social interpretation.

The Unemployment Conundrum

Consider the journey of a highly capable individual entering the workforce, perhaps a recent graduate or a mid-career professional. On paper, they are brilliant: Analytical, detail-oriented, and deeply committed to accuracy. But in practice, they struggle. Not with the work itself but with the invisible architecture of the workplace; the unspoken rules, shifting expectations, and subtle social hierarchies that govern professional environments.

Traditional models might explain these difficulties through theories such as Executive Dysfunction Theory or ToM, suggesting deficits – in predicting others, planning, flexibility, or multitasking. Others might point to a lack of social motivation or emotional intelligence. However, Mind Fidelity Theory offers a more integrated and compassionate explanation.

In high-fidelity perception and cognition, the brain favors deliberate, logical, and effortful Type 2 processing. This mode of thinking excels in structured problem-solving and deep focus, but it comes at a cost: It consumes significant cognitive resources. As a result, there's less bandwidth available for rapid context-switching, intuitive social inference, or adapting to vague instructions. What looks like inflexibility or poor time management is often the result of a mind already operating at full capacity, prioritizing accuracy over performance speed.

This same cognitive architecture also resists the short-cuts and biases that most people unconsciously rely on to navigate social situations. Neurotypical individuals often use heuristics, like the halo effect, authority bias, or emotional mirroring, to make quick judgments and build rapport. But a high-fidelity mind doesn't default to these. It seeks clarity, not consensus. It values truth over tact. And in a workplace where social cohesion often trumps objective accuracy, this can lead to friction.

For example, a high-fidelity thinker might question a vague directive from a manager, not out of defiance but out of a genuine need for clarity. They might point out inconsistencies in a team's strategy, not to undermine but to improve it. Yet these actions, stripped of the expected social framing, can be misinterpreted as blunt, difficult, or even insubordinate.

Over time, this mismatch can lead to social breakdowns, strained relationships, missed promotions, or even job losses. The individual may reflect on a career marked by frequent transitions, interpersonal stress, and a persistent sense of not quite fitting in. But the issue isn't a lack of competence or motivation. It's a fundamental difference in how reality is processed and prioritized.

In this light, what appears to be executive dysfunction or social detachment is better understood as a cognitive trade-off. The same fidelity that drives analytical brilliance can make social navigation more effortful. The absence of bias, while intellectually powerful, can leave a person vulnerable in environments that reward emotional fluency over logical integrity. It can also lead to treating others as they truly are, rather than as they are socially perceived – an approach that may clash with group expectations. Because high-fidelity thinkers do not intuitively grasp the socially constructed illusions others operate under, such as the halo effect, they cannot easily mask or mimic those perceptions, making their authenticity both a strength and a social liability.

These lived experiences illustrate how the diagnostic criteria for autism can be reinterpreted through the lens of Mind Fidelity Theory. Rather than viewing autistic traits solely as deficits in communication, flexibility, or social motivation, this framework suggests the deficits identified in diagnostic criteria are simply differences in how a mind perceives reality in tune with the social construct of the human environment.

But what happens when the environment shifts such as the environmental complexity we now face? Where, then, does the deficit and disability lie?

Imagine you're in the courtroom. You must choose between two judges, one autistic, who relies on logic and consistency, and one neurotypical, whose decisions may be shaped by intuition, emotion, and social norms. In a world growing more complex and data-driven, the autistic judge may offer a more stable and impartial perspective – less swayed by bias, more anchored in evidence.

This scenario illustrates a key principle of Mind Fidelity Theory: As environments become more abstract and interconnected, traits once seen as deficits may become assets. Autism, with its emphasis on precision and pattern recognition, offers a cognitive style better suited to navigating complexity.

However, not all autistic traits align perfectly with this shift. Some may still pose challenges in highly social or ambiguous contexts. But the point remains; disability should not be measured against the majority, but against the cognitive profile best equipped to meet the demands of the environment.

ASD 1, 2, 3

Imagine a radio picking up every station at once – music, news, static, voices – without the ability to tune in or filter. For some individuals with Level 3 autism, this may be how the world is experienced: All sensory input is received, but without the neural filtering that assigns meaning or context. At this most profound level of the spectrum, Mind Fidelity Theory suggests that individuals may experience a form of cognitive disconnection – not from the world, but from their own internal processing. Rather than being overwhelmed by external stimuli alone, they may also struggle to access or organize their own thoughts, due to reduced top-down processing and enhanced Type 2 thinking, making communication and interaction profoundly challenging.

This cognitive profile results in a profound difficulty organizing information into coherent structures, or filter it based on relevance or context. The brain, in this state, may process each new input with such literal accuracy that it lacks the associative framework needed for intuitive understanding or flexible response. In essence, the mind becomes a high-fidelity receiver with no internal compression algorithm; everything is taken in, but little is synthesized.

As the minds fidelity decreases, moving toward Level 2 and Level 1 presentations of autism, the ability to perceive and interpret internally improves, though often through conscious, effortful processing rather than intuitive flow. Social behaviors, emotional interpretations, and contextual understanding may emerge, but they are often constructed deliberately rather than arising automatically.

John Etherington

As stabilizing selection shapes human cognition in response to the modern world, where information is abundant, contradictions are frequent, and discerning truth is more valuable than passive acceptance, the extreme traits associated with autism may gradually soften.

In this context, the severity of autistic traits may lessen, not due to elimination, but because the cognitive strengths they offer are becoming more integrated into the broader population. Thus, an increase in those diagnosed with autistic traits.

This perspective reframes autism not as a spectrum of impairment, but as a spectrum of perception and cognitive configurations shared across the human population. It highlights a fundamental trade-off between fidelity to objective reality and social flexibility, one that shapes how individuals perceive, process, and respond to the world around them.

As we've seen, Mind Fidelity Theory offers a powerful new lens through which to understand the behaviors and experiences that define autism, not as signs of dysfunction but as expressions of a different cognitive architecture. But this reframing raises a deeper question: What does it mean for the future of humanity?

If autistic traits reflect a mind better suited to navigating complexity by resisting bias and seeking truth in a world of noise, and as a species, we are adapting to this new world with higher levels of perceptive and cognitive fidelity to objective reality, identified as autistic traits, what does this mean for our species as a whole?

To explore this question, we will use Plato's Allegory of the Cave as a canvas, touched on earlier in the book.

CHAPTER 10: LEAVING THE CAVE — HUMANITY'S NEXT STEP

For millennia, we have lived in a world of shadows. Plato's Allegory of the Cave, written over 2,000 years ago, tells the story of prisoners chained in a dark cavern facing a wall.

Behind them, a fire casts shadows of objects carried by unseen figures. To the prisoners, these shadows are reality. They know nothing else. One day, a prisoner is freed. He stumbles into the light, overwhelmed by its brilliance. At first, he resists it. But slowly, his eyes adjust. He sees the world as it truly is, not as shadows but in full color and form. When he returns to the cave to share what he's seen, the others reject him. They mock him. Some even threaten him.

This allegory has been interpreted in many ways: As a metaphor for education or enlightenment, or as the painful process of confronting truth. But at its core, it is a story about perception and the resistance we face when that perception is challenged.

The Cave as Cognitive Illusion

In the modern world, the cave is not a place. It is a state of mind.

The shackles are not chains of iron but of belief bias, cognitive shortcuts, and inherited assumptions. The shadows are not cast by puppeteers but by our own brains, constructing reality from fragments of experience filtered through memory, emotion, and expectation.

Most of us live in this cave without knowing it. We trust our perceptions because they feel real. We believe what we see, hear, and think, even when those beliefs are shaped more by social consensus than by objective truth.

But what if some minds are born outside the cave?

The Unshackled Mind

Mind Fidelity Theory proposes that autistic traits are caused by high-fidelity perception and cognition that processes the world/reality with less distortion. These minds rely less on internal filters and more on raw sensory input. They are less swayed by social framing, more attuned to inconsistencies, and more committed to accuracy over assumption.

In Plato's allegory, the freed prisoner is overwhelmed by the light. He struggles to make sense of a world that contradicts everything he once believed. This mirrors the experience of many autistic individuals, who also struggle to make sense of the world not because they are broken, but because they are perceiving more, in more detail, and in more complexity, resulting in more truth.

Like the freed prisoner, they are often misunderstood. Their insights are dismissed. Their differences are pathologized. They are told to return to the cave, to conform, to mask, to pretend.

But what if they are not the ones who need to change?

A Species at the Threshold

Humanity is growing up. For centuries, we have lived by inherited rules, moral codes, and simplified worldviews. These were our training wheels, the scaffolding that helped us survive in a world of scarcity, danger, and tribal conflict. But the world has changed. We no longer face the same dangers we once required protection from. Our main threat is now ourselves, not from what's outside the cave but from what's within.

We now live in a world of accelerating complexity, a world shaped by global networks, artificial intelligence, climate change, and cultural pluralism. The shadows on the wall no longer suffice. The old shortcuts, intuition, conformity, and beliefs are breaking down.

We are at a threshold. Like a young adult leaving home, we are stepping into the unknown. The light is bright. It stings our eyes. But it is also beautiful and offers a new way forward.

The Evolution of Perception

Mind Fidelity Theory suggests that this transition is not just cultural; it is biological. As our environment becomes more complex, evolution may be favoring minds that can process reality with greater fidelity. Minds that resist illusion. Minds that question assumptions. Minds that see clearly, even when it hurts.

These minds may not fit easily into traditional systems. They often show little interest in small talk, office politics, or the social games that define status within the cave. It's not that they can't play; it's that they see no value in the game. Competing over shadows, climbing invisible ladders, or seeking approval from those still shackled simply doesn't matter when you've glimpsed the world beyond. For those who have tasted the clarity of the light, the goals and judgments of the cave lose their meaning. Their attention turns outward to patterns, to truth, to the vast and intricate reality that lies beyond the wall. These individuals are not defective. They are different. And in a world that demands clarity, they may be the ones best equipped to lead.

The New Light

Leaving the cave is not easy. It requires courage. It requires letting go of comforting illusions. It requires facing the discomfort of not knowing and the responsibility of seeing.

But it also offers something extraordinary: The chance to build a new world. A world not based on shadows but on substance. Not on conformity, but on truth. Not on illusion but on insight.

In this new world, the unshackled minds are not outcasts. They are guides. They are the ones who have already seen the light and who can help the rest of us find our way.

Beyond the Cave: Minds Drawn to the Light

We are no longer prisoners. The chains are loosening. The wall is cracking. The light is spilling in.

But this is not a single moment of awakening; it is a transition. A slow, uneven emergence from illusion into clarity. Not all minds experience this shift in the same way.

Imagine a mind so far beyond the cave that it has never known the shadows. A mind immersed in raw, unfiltered reality, where all sound, light, and sensation arrive with full intensity. Mind Fidelity Theory proposes this is the experience of someone with Level 3 autism. Not broken, but lost, and so deeply attuned to the world beyond the cave that the rituals and rules of those still inside are not just irrelevant, they are inaccessible. These individuals are oriented toward a different kind of perception, an extreme evolutionary hedge, one that does not pass through subconscious filters and does not organize the senses from memory and experience.

Now imagine a mind that lives at the edge of the cave's reach, close enough to see the shadows but far enough that they never quite make sense. This is the experience of Level 2 autism. These individuals may attempt to engage with the world of the cave, but the interactions are often brief, confusing, or strained. The logic of the shadows, the games of status, and the unspoken rules are too abstract to recognize. Their insights are often missed, and their presence is misunderstood.

And then there are those with Level 1 autism, minds that can come and go. They can enter the cave, observe the shadows, and even mimic the movements of those still shackled. But they do not stay. They do not invest in the game. The shadows hold no power over them because they have seen what casts them. They know the source. And once you've seen the fire or the sun beyond it, the flickering illusions on the wall lose their meaning. These minds are not interested in climbing the social ladder or winning arguments about the shadows. Not because they can't, but because they see no value in doing so. Their attention is drawn to the light, the patterns, the systems, and the truths that lie beyond the cave.

This is the spectrum of perception and cognition. And it is also the spectrum of our future.

Final Reflection: The Light Ahead

Humanity is at a threshold. We are stepping out of the cave, not all at once, and not all in the same way. But the direction is clear. The complexity of our world demands minds that can see beyond illusion, that can resist belief and bias, and that can process reality with greater fidelity.

These minds may not fit easily into traditional systems, but they are not here to fit in. They are here to show us where we are heading and what lies beyond.

We are evolving, not away from our past, but through it. We are learning to see not just what is expected but what is real. And as we step into the light, blinking in the brightness of a new dawn, we may finally begin to understand.

The future does not belong to those who master the shadows.

It belongs to those who have the courage to leave them behind, and the vision to build something new in the light.

FINAL SUMMARY: THE CAUSE OF AUTISM THROUGH MIND FIDELITY THEORY

Mind Fidelity Theory proposes that human perception and cognition exist on a spectrum of fidelity to objective reality. This spectrum reflects both individual variation and broader evolutionary trends across the human population. In this framework, autism is not a disorder but a manifestation of heightened perceptual and cognitive fidelity – an increased alignment with external reality and reduced reliance on internal filters such as bias, expectation, and social framing.

As human environments have grown more complex – driven by globalization, digital systems, and information density – the cognitive demands placed on individuals have shifted. In such environments, greater accuracy in perception and reasoning becomes increasingly advantageous. This shift creates evolutionary pressure favoring traits that support veridical (truth-aligned) perception and cognition.

Through the process of stabilizing selection, genes that enhance perceptual fidelity are becoming more prevalent in the human gene pool. These genetic changes influence the sensory and cognitive systems, increasing access to raw, unfiltered reality. However, this comes with trade-offs: reduced internal organization, diminished reliance on social heuristics, and increased cognitive load. These trade-offs manifest behaviorally along a spectrum – from subtle traits to profound differences – mirroring the diverse presentations of autism.

Autism, therefore, is not caused by dysfunction, but by biological adaptation to a rapidly evolving environment. The increasing complexity of our world is selecting for minds that resist illusion, prioritize logic, and perceive reality with greater clarity. Autistic traits are the cognitive signatures of this adaptation.

In this view, autism is not a deviation from the norm, but a signal of where human cognition is heading.

ABOUT THE AUTHOR

In 2015, after a lifetime of challenges in education and employment, John Etherington was formally diagnosed with autism. The diagnosis brought clarity to a journey long marked by misunderstanding, misalignment, and a persistent sense of being out of step with the systems around him. Yet, despite these challenges, he achieved academic success and rose to executive-level leadership in the fields of digital engineering and spatial science.

Throughout his career, he has designed and implemented large-scale project systems for teams exceeding 120 staff, more than 80 of whom were autistic. In this environment, he witnessed firsthand the profound disconnect between neurotypical expectations and the cognitive realities of autistic individuals. Even at the executive level, he encountered resistance, bias, and a deep-rooted misunderstanding of how different minds perceive and process the world.

These experiences led him to question the prevailing models of autism and to explore a new framework, one that could account not only for the challenges autistic individuals face but also for the unique strengths they bring. This exploration became the foundation of what he now calls Mind Fidelity Theory.

In recent years, researchers across disciplines have called for a unified theory of autism, one that bridges the gaps between psychology, neuroscience, systems theory, and lived experience. The author's current PhD research is a direct response to that call. He is developing interdisciplinary models that integrate cognitive science, artificial intelligence, and organizational design to better understand communication strategies between individuals with varying levels of cognitive fidelity, particularly in the workplace, where these differences often go unrecognized or unsupported.

This book is a glimpse into that research. It is both a theoretical framework and a practical guide, a bridge between philosophy, neuroscience, and systems thinking. It is written not only for those who seek to understand autism but for anyone interested in how human cognition is evolving in response to an increasingly complex world.

REFERENCES

1. Harvery, M., et al., *Employment profiles of autistic adults in Australia.* Autism research : official journal of the International Society for Autism Research, 2021. **14**(10): p. 2061–2077.
2. Sandra Jones, M.A., Nicole Murphy, Paul Myers and a.N. Vickers, *Employment, Community Attitudes, and Lived Experiences Research Report.* 2019: Amaze.com.
3. Mavranezouli, I., et al., *The cost-effectiveness of supported employment for adults with autism in the United Kingdom.* Autism, 2014. **18**(8): p. 975-984.
4. Solomon, C., *Autism and Employment: Implications for Employers and Adults with ASD.* Journal of Autism and Developmental Disorders, 2020. **50**(11): p. 4209–4217.
5. Wen, B., et al., *Autism and neurodiversity in the workplace: A scoping review of key trends, employer roles, interventions and supports.* Journal of Vocational Rehabilitation, 2023. **60**(1): p. 121–140.
6. Sivakumar, V., et al., *Phantom vibration and ringing syndromes among Indian medical students.* Bioinformation, 2024. **20**(8): p. 842–848.
7. Thériault, R., M. Landry, and A. Raz, *The Rubber Hand*

Illusion: Top-down attention modulates embodiment. Quarterly Journal of Experimental Psychology, 2022. **75**(11): p. 2129–2148.
8. St B. T. Evans, J. and K.E. Stanovich, *Dual-Process Theories of Higher Cognition: Advancing the Debate.* Perspectives on Psychological Science, 2013. **8**(3): p. 223-241.
9. Holyoak, K.J. and R.G. Morrison, *The Oxford handbook of thinking and reasoning.* 2012, Oxford University Press: New York.
10. Brosnan, M., M. Lewton, and C. Ashwin, *Reasoning on the Autism Spectrum: A Dual Process Theory Account.* Journal of autism and developmental disorders, 2016. **46**(6): p. 2115–2125.
11. Feinstein, A., *A history of autism : conversations with the pioneers.* 2010, Wiley-Blackwell: Chichester, West Sussex, United Kingdom.
12. Lyons, V. and M. Fitzgerald, *Asperger (1906-1980) and Kanner (1894-1981), the two pioneers of autism.* Journal of autism and developmental disorders, 2007. **37**(10): p. 2022-3.
13. Pasco, G., *The diagnosis and epidemiology of autism.* Tizard Learning Disability Review, 2011. **16**(4): p. 5–19.
14. Regier, D.A., E.A. Kuhl, and D.J. Kupfer, *The DSM-5: Classification and criteria changes.* World Psychiatry, 2013. **12**(2): p. 92-98.
15. Grant, C.M., A. Grayson, and J. Boucher, *Using Tests of False Belief with Children with Autism: How Valid and Reliable are they?* Autism, 2001. **5**(2): p. 135–145.
16. Happé, F. and U. Frith, *The Weak Coherence Account: Detail-focused Cognitive Style in Autism Spectrum Disorders.* Journal of Autism and Developmental

Disorders, 2006. **36**(1): p. 5-25.
17. Demetriou, E.A., M.M. DeMayo, and A.J. Guastella, *Executive Function in Autism Spectrum Disorder: History, Theoretical Models, Empirical Findings, and Potential as an Endophenotype.* Frontiers in psychiatry, 2019. **10**: p. 753.
18. Milton, D.E.M., *On the ontological status of autism: the 'double empathy problem'.* Disability & Society, 2012. **27**(6): p. 883–887.
19. Southey, S., et al., *Autistic Perspectives on Employment: A Scoping Review.* Journal of occupational rehabilitation, 2024. **34**(4): p. 756–769.
20. Mark, J.T., B.B. Marion, and D.D. Hoffman, *Natural selection and veridical perceptions.* Journal of theoretical biology, 2010. **266**(4): p. 504–15.
21. Hansen, T.F., *STABILIZING SELECTION AND THE COMPARATIVE ANALYSIS OF ADAPTATION.* Evolution, 1997. **51**(5): p. 1341–1351.
22. Grinin, L., *Periodization of history: a theoretic-mathematical analysis.* History and mathematics: Analyzing and modeling global development, 2006: p. 10–38.
23. Morsanyi, K. and R. Byrne, *Thinking, Reasoning, and Decision Making in Autism.* 2019, Routledge: Milton.
24. Rozenkrantz, L., A.M. D'Mello, and J.D.E. Gabrieli, *Enhanced rationality in autism spectrum disorder.* Trends in Cognitive Sciences, 2021. **25**(8): p. 685–696.
25. van der Plas, E., D. Mason, and F. Happé, *Decision-making in autism: A narrative review.* Autism, 2023.
26. Soulières, I., et al., *Enhanced visual processing contributes to matrix reasoning in autism.* Human brain mapping, 2009. **30**(12): p. 4082–107.

27. Brosnan, M. and C. Ashwin, *Thinking, fast and slow on the autism spectrum.* Autism : the international journal of research and practice, 2023. **27**(5): p. 1245–1255.
28. Robertson, C.E. and S. Baron-Cohen, *Sensory perception in autism.* Nature reviews. Neuroscience, 2017. **18**(11): p. 671–684.
29. Marco, E.J., et al., *Sensory processing in autism: a review of neurophysiologic findings.* Pediatric research, 2011. **69**(5 Pt 2): p. 48R-54R.
30. Tomasi, D. and N.D. Volkow, *Reduced Local and Increased Long-Range Functional Connectivity of the Thalamus in Autism Spectrum Disorder.* Cerebral Cortex, 2019. **29**(2): p. 573–585.
31. Baran, B., et al., *Increased resting-state thalamocortical functional connectivity in children and young adults with autism spectrum disorder.* Autism research : official journal of the International Society for Autism Research, 2023. **16**(2): p. 271–279.
32. Ursino, M., et al., *Bottom-up vs. top-down connectivity imbalance in individuals with high-autistic traits: An electroencephalographic study.* Frontiers in Systems Neuroscience, 2022. **16**.
33. Harmon-Jones, E., *Cognitive dissonance : reexamining a pivotal theory in psychology.* 2019, American Psychological Association: Washington, DC.
34. Kaplan, J.T., S.I. Gimbel, and S. Harris, *Neural correlates of maintaining one's political beliefs in the face of counterevidence.* Scientific reports, 2016. **6**: p. 39589.
35. Sebat, J., et al., *Strong Association of De Novo Copy Number Mutations with Autism.* Science, 2007. **316**(5823): p. 445–449.
36. Rodriguez-Gomez, D.A., et al. *A systematic review of*

common genetic variation and biological pathways in autism spectrum disorder. BMC Neuroscience, 2021. **22**, DOI: 10.1186/s12868-021-00662-z.
37. Constantino, J., et al. *Sex and gender differences in autism spectrum disorder: summarizing evidence gaps and identifying emerging areas of priority.* Molecular Autism, 2015. **6**, 1-5 DOI: 10.1186/s13229-015-0019-y.
38. Pollard, K.S., et al., *An RNA gene expressed during cortical development evolved rapidly in humans.* Nature, 2006. **443**(7108): p. 167–72.
39. Doan, R.N., et al., *Mutations in Human Accelerated Regions (HARs) Disrupt Cognition and Social Behavior.* Cell, 2016. **167**(2): p. 341–354.e12.
40. Sanjak, J.S., et al., *Evidence of directional and stabilizing selection in contemporary humans.* Proceedings of the National Academy of Sciences, 2018. **115**(1): p. 151–156.
41. Premack, D. and G. Woodruff, *Does the chimpanzee have a theory of mind?* Behavioral and Brain Sciences, 1978. **1**(4): p. 515–526.
42. Frith, U. and F. Happé, *Autism: beyond "theory of mind".* Cognition, 1994. **50**(1-3): p. 115–32.
43. Chevallier, C., et al., *The social motivation theory of autism.* Trends in cognitive sciences, 2012. **16**(4): p. 231–9.
44. Uljarević, M., et al., *Challenges to the social motivation theory of autism: The dangers of counteracting an imprecise theory with even more imprecision.* Behavioral and Brain Sciences, 2019. **42**.
45. Qin, L., et al., *New advances in the diagnosis and treatment of autism spectrum disorders.* European journal of medical research, 2024. **29**(1): p. 322.

www.ingramcontent.com/pod-product-compliance
Lightning Source LLC
Chambersburg PA
CBHW060031040426
42333CB00042B/2310